GUIDE TO

Rhythmically Moving

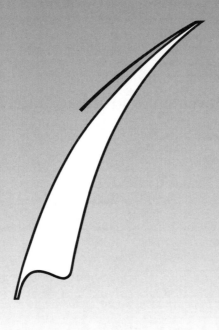

Related Movement and Music Materials

Available from

High/Scope Press

600 North River Street, Ypsilanti, Michigan 48198-2898
ORDERS: phone (800)40-PRESS, fax (800)422-4FAX

GUIDE TO

Rhythmically Moving

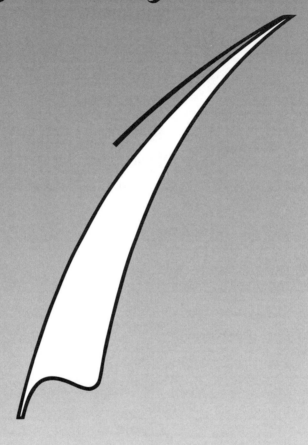

Elizabeth B. Carlton
Phyllis S. Weikart

HIGH/SCOPE PRESS
YPSILANTI, MICHIGAN

Published by
THE HIGH/SCOPE PRESS
A division of
High/Scope Educational Research Foundation
600 North River Street
Ypsilanti, Michigan 48198-2898
313/485-2000, FAX 313/485-0704

Editor: Marge Senninger
Design and layout: Margaret FitzGerald

ISBN 1-57379-004-4

Printed in the United States of America
10 9 8 7 6 5 4 3 2 1

CONTENTS

The *Rhythmically Moving* series of nine recordings is a rare collection of international folk music that can have a major impact on students as they learn to develop basic timing and musicianship. Besides providing the music for the folk dances notated in *Teaching Movement & Dance: A Sequential Approach to Rhythmic Movement*, Third Edition, the recordings can be used to introduce or reinforce the movement and music concepts described in two related publications, *Foundations in Elementary Education: Music* and *Foundations in Elementary Education: Movement*. The music is also used with other print and video products of the High/Scope Press.

This guide will help you receive the maximum benefit from the first of the *Rhythmically Moving* recordings (RM1). Using the information included here, you can help students to understand and grow through the music on this recording as they listen, move, dance, sing, play instruments, relate ideas, and become personally involved with particular melodies and harmonies. Some students will be interested in identifying the predominant instrument in a selection; others may want to learn the melody, so they can respond to its mood another day; still others may want to play the melody or "chord along" on an autoharp or guitar while others sing. In a consistent format, this guide provides all the information that is needed to facilitate the many and varied activities necessary for students' understanding and application of movement and music concepts.

For each selection, you will find the **title,** the **band** on which the selection can be found, the overall **length** in minutes and seconds, and the national or regional **origin** of the selection. We also indicate whether the selection is **vocal or instrumental** and the **major instruments** played. The **number of repetitions of the selection** is also noted. More specialized information, such as the following, is included:

- **Melodic form:** The musical phrases (abcd) or musical sections (AABB, ABC) are identified, and when appropriate, the selection is described as a round (or canon), a rondo, or a theme and variations.

- **Beat:** The number of **microbeats or macrobeats in the introduction** to the selection is noted, as correlated with the stepping beat of the dance. (The terms *microbeat* and *macrobeat* are Dr. Edwin Gordon's terms.)

- **Tempo:** The per-minute pace of the macrobeats or microbeats is also indicated.

- **Meter:** We indicate if the microbeats are grouped in twos (duple meter) or threes (triple meter).

- **Key or mode:** For most selections, we indicate the tonal center, as determined by the scale (major or minor) and the key signature at the beginning of the music notation. For some selections, we identify the modality (such as D Dorian or G Mixolydian).

- **Traditional music notation with key (or mode), time signature, and primary chords identified:** For each selection, we provide the **notated melody** within the **rhythmic framework** indicated by the time signature. This provides melodic examples that you may want to excerpt for use as dictation exercises for advanced students. Students can also use the musical notation to see how durational relationships are represented as they experience the rhythm of the recording. Rhythmic examples may be excerpted for use as rhythmic puzzles for students to decode or as rhythmic dictation challenges. In the musical notation, **primary chords** are shown above the melody as A (for A major), Em (for E minor), D⁷, etc. A chord symbol such as "G/D" indicates a G major chord is used with a D as the lowest tone played. Roman numerals below the melody also indicate the chords based on the given key system.

To assist you in coordinating the musical selections on RM1 with content in related books or videos, this guide also lists the important **music concepts** to be identified in each selection, as well as the important **movement concepts for dance** (the specific concepts relating to the folk dance associated with the musical selection).

A list of **suggestions for use** is also given. This list usually contains page citations from the **related books** *Movement Plus Music, Foundations in Elementary Education: Music,* and *Foundations in Elementary Education: Movement.* In connection with these latter two books, we also provide a list of relevant key experiences in movement and music. Also included in the **suggestions for use** are **activities** in music and movement that "fit" the particular musical selection.

If the selection corresponds to a **folk dance** taught in the book *Teaching Movement and Dance: A Sequential Approach,* this is indicated, along with the page number on which you can find the steps for teaching the folk dance. Likewise, if the selection is demonstrated on one of High/Scope's *Beginning Folk Dances Illustrated* videotapes, this information is also provided.

The **additional information** about each selection may tell you more about the title, the origin or composer, the sections or phrasing, or other items of interest.

The wealth of information contained in this guide will enable you to use the *Rhythmically Moving 1* recording to help students make connections to a wide variety of music and movement concepts. As students begin to understand and apply these concepts, they will develop a music and movement foundation that can only grow stronger throughout life.

ALL THE WAY TO GALWAY

Band: 1

Origin: Ireland

Melodic form: AABB

Type of selection: Instrumental

Introduction: 4 microbeats

Length: 1:51

Meter: Duple

Key or mode: E-flat major

Major instrument(s): Piano, penny-whistle, violin

Tempo: 146 microbeats per minute

Repetitions of selection: 4

Music concepts

Steady beat, same/different melodic phrases, form, melodic variation, *allegro* tempo, primary chord progression patterns, D.S. (return to the sign, 𝄋)

Movement concepts for dance

Steady beat, directionality, nonlocomotor/locomotor movement, personal/general space

Suggestions for use

With related books

Movement Plus Music, p. 7

Foundations in Elementary Education: Music, work with these key experiences in music:

- Moving to music
- Feeling and expressing steady beat
- Labeling form
- Recognizing the expressive qualities of tempo
- Feeling and identifying meter

Foundations in Elementary Education: Movement, work with these key experiences in movement:

- Acting upon movement directions
- Feeling and expressing steady beat
- Moving in sequences to a common beat

In activities

Perform aerobic fitness routines.

Participate in jogging parades with four students in each line; pause to change leaders on each repetition of selection.

Lead static Stages of Movement for Responding, changing every 8 beats.

Folk dance

Teaching Movement & Dance: A Sequential Approach (Two-Part Dance), p. 142

Additional information

During the third and fourth repetitions, a melodic variation occurs in the second phrase of the A section.

There is a piano vamp in the introduction.

Melodic notation with primary chords identified

(see next page)

All the Way to Galway

Irish Melody

Intro.

Allegro

A Section

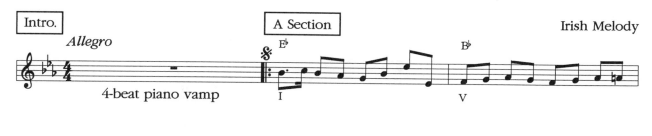

4-beat piano vamp

B Section

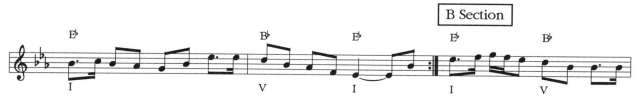

1.

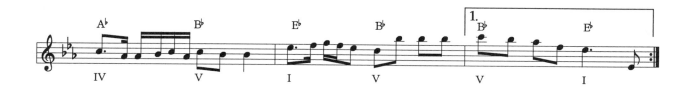

2.

* *D. S.*

Final Ending

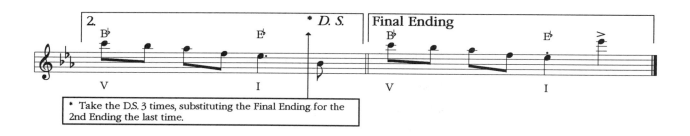

> * Take the D.S. 3 times, substituting the Final Ending for the 2nd Ending the last time.

SLIDING

Band: 2	
Origin: United States	**Meter:** Duple
Melodic form: aabbcc (phrases)	**Key or mode:** G major
Type of selection: Instrumental	**Major instrument(s):** Guitar
Introduction: 8 microbeats	**Tempo:** 128 microbeats per minute
Length: 1:41	**Repetitions of selection:** 4

Music concepts

Steady beat; repetition; same/different melodic phrases; form; syncopation; *staccato;* repeated chord progression pattern: I, I, IV, I

Movement concepts for dance

Steady beat, recurring 2-beat nonlocomotor movement sequence, same/different pathways, personal/general space

Suggestions for use

With related books

Foundations in Elementary Education: Music, pp. 67, 103; also work with these key experiences in music:

- Moving to music
- Feeling and expressing steady beat
- Labeling form
- Responding to various types of music

Foundations in Elementary Education: Movement, p. 284; also work with these key experiences in movement:

- Acting upon movement directions
- Feeling and expressing steady beat
- Moving in sequences to a common beat

In activities

Rock with the macrobeat.

Choose three ways to twist, swing, turn, etc. for the three sections of the music.

Perform three locomotor movements for the three sections of the music.

Bounce and catch a ball (alone or with a partner) on the macrobeat.

Develop passing patterns for beanbags or lumee sticks on the macrobeat.

Lead movement echo sequences.

Encourage students to listen for melody patterns, phrases, primary chords, form, and instrument identification.

Folk dance

Teaching Movement & Dance: A Sequential Approach, p. 140

Additional information:

Sliding is composed by Sandor Slomovits and performed by Gemini.

A guitar countermelody is played during the second and fourth repetitions.

The dance is choreographed by Phyllis S. Weikart.

Melodic notation with primary chords identified

(see next page)

Sliding

American Melody
Composed by Sandor Slomovits

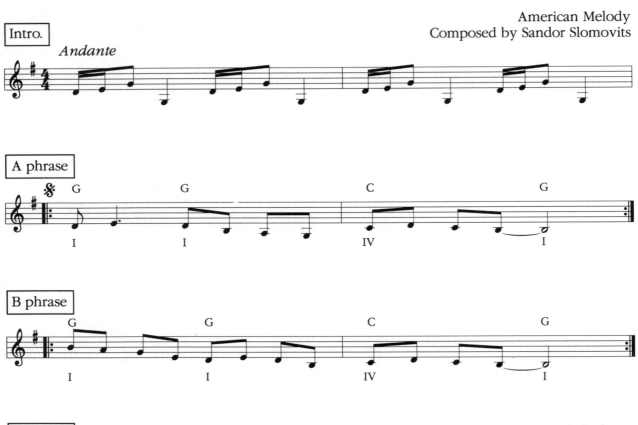

* Take the D.S. 3 times, thus playing the entire melody 4 times.

BRIAN BORU'S MARCH

Band: 3

Origin: Ireland

Melodic form: AABB

Type of selection: Instrumental

Introduction: 4 microbeats

Length: 2:11

Meter: Duple

Key or mode: A Aeolian modality or A pure minor

Major instrument(s): Violin, guitar

Tempo: 82 microbeats per minute

Repetitions of selection: 2½ + *coda*

Music concepts

Steady beat, phrase, *coda*, melodic sequences, microbeat divided into three, repetition of rhythmic patterns, *moderato* tempo, *ritardando*, 8va, D.S. (return to the sign, 𝄋)

Suggestions for use

With related books

Movement Plus Music, pp. 22, 38

Foundations in Elementary Education: Music, work with these key experiences in music:

- ⚷ Moving to music
- ⚷ Feeling and expressing steady beat
- ⚷ Labeling form
- ⚷ Feeling and identifying meter
- ⚷ Responding to various types of music

Foundations in Elementary Education: Movement, work with these key experiences in movement:

- ⚷ Acting upon movement directions
- ⚷ Feeling and expressing steady beat
- ⚷ Moving in sequences to a common beat

In activities

Practice ball routines (bounce/catch, toss/catch).

Perform routines with beanbags or lumee sticks.

Move creatively with scarves.

Lead movement echo sequences.

Lead alternated sequences (Levels V and VI of Beat Coordination).

Skate to the macrobeat.

Conduct in a two-beat conductor's pattern.

Lead slow dynamic movements for mirroring or reversal.

Folk dance

None

Additional information

During the second repetition, the violin plays the melody one octave higher.

Melodic notation with primary chords identified

(see next page)

Brian Boru's March

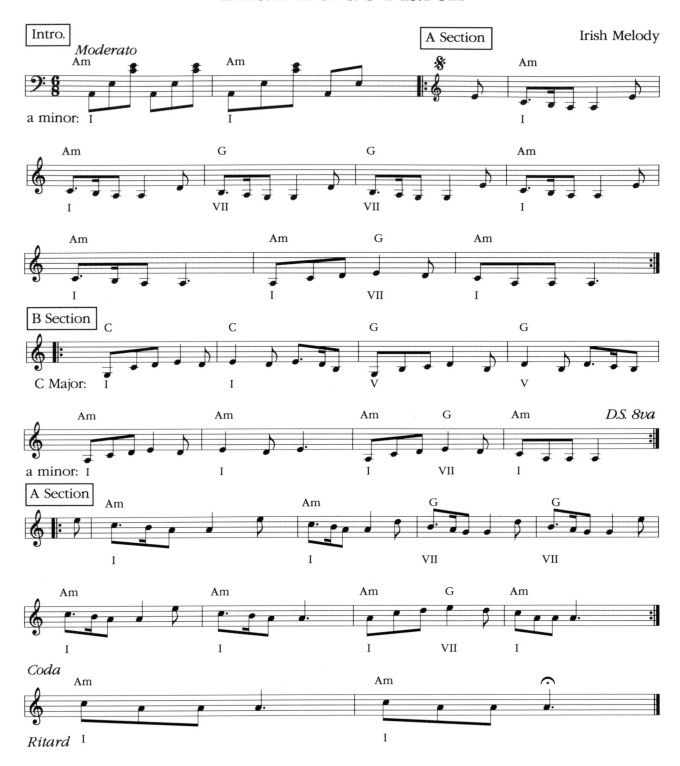

HAPPY FEET

Band: 4	
Origin: United States	**Meter:** Duple
Melodic form: AABB	**Key or mode:** E-flat major
Type of selection: Instrumental	**Major instrument(s):** Violin, guitar
Introduction: 4 microbeats	**Tempo:** 100 microbeats per minute
Length: 2:04	**Repetitions of selection:** 3

Music concepts

Steady beat; rhythm patterns using sixteenth notes; form; *moderato* tempo; *staccato;* melodic and rhythmic dictation; I, V chord identification, D.S. (return to the sign, $\mathcal{S}$)

Suggestions for use

With related books

Movement Plus Music, p. 38

Foundations in Elementary Education: Music, work with these key experiences in music:

- Moving to music
- Labeling form
- Writing music
- Developing melody
- Responding to various types of music
- Moving creatively

Foundations in Elementary Education: Movement, p. 223; also work with these key experiences in movement:

- Moving in nonlocomotor ways
- Moving in locomotor ways
- Moving with objects
- Feeling and expressing steady beat
- Expressing creativity in movement

In activities

Perform aerobic routines.

Represent action words, such as *dab, flick,* to the music.

Practice ball skills (bounce/catch, pass, dribble) to the music.

Represent the concept of "happy" with hands, feet, and other body parts.

Represent movements of robots, clowns, etc.

Participate in jogging parades.

Folk dance

None

Additional information

Happy Feet is composed by Laszlo Slomovits and performed by Gemini.

During the second and third repetitions, the melody is played one octave lower.

Melodic notation with primary chords identified

(see next page)

Happy Feet

American Melody
Composed by Laszlo Slomovits

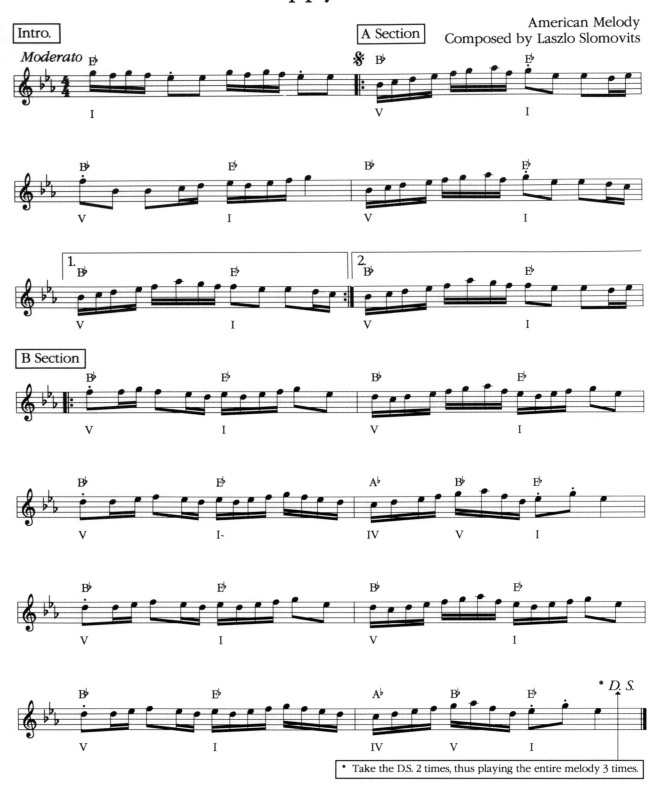

* Take the D.S. 2 times, thus playing the entire melody 3 times.

OH, HOW LOVELY

Band: 5

Origin: England

Melodic form: abc (phrases), canon

Type of selection: Instrumental

Introduction: 4 macrobeats

Length: 1:44

Meter: Triple

Key or mode: D major

Major instrument(s): Violin, guitar, recorder

Tempo: 66 macrobeats per minute, 198 microbeats per minute

Repetitions of selection: 5

Music concepts

Steady macrobeat; long and short phrases; melodic sequences; round or canon; *ritardando*; repeated chord patterns: I, I, IV, I, IV, I; D.S. (return to the sign, 𝄋)

Movement concepts for dance

Directionality of forward, sideward, backward; canon movement; movement to the macrobeat

Suggestions for use

With related books

Movement Plus Music, pp. 28, 36

Foundations in Elementary Education: Music, p. 285; also work with these key experiences in music:

- Moving to music
- Feeling and expressing steady beat
- Developing melody
- Labeling form
- Feeling and identifying meter
- Adding harmony

Foundations in Elementary Education: Movement, p. 175; also work with these key experiences in movement:

- Moving in nonlocomotor ways
- Moving in locomotor ways

- Moving with objects
- Expressing creativity
- Feeling and expressing steady beat
- Moving in sequences to a common beat

In activities

Lead canon movement to the music.

Practice rocking, swinging, and turning movements.

Move creatively with scarves, ribbon wands, paper plates.

Lead slow dynamic movements for copycat or mirroring.

Walk or skate to the macrobeat.

Practice ball skills (toss/catch, bounce/catch).

Pass beanbags to the macrobeat.

Play tonebar instruments on the macrobeat (pentatonic setup).

Folk dance

Teaching Movement & Dance: A Sequential Approach, p. 164

Additional information

The third and fourth phrases are sequences of the first and second phrases.

The D is the common tone in both the I chord (D, F♯, A) and the IV chord (G, B, D), therefore this single tone can be played as a simple macrobeat accompaniment.

The dance is choreographed by Phyllis S. Weikart.

Melodic notation with primary chords identified

(see next page)

Oh, How Lovely

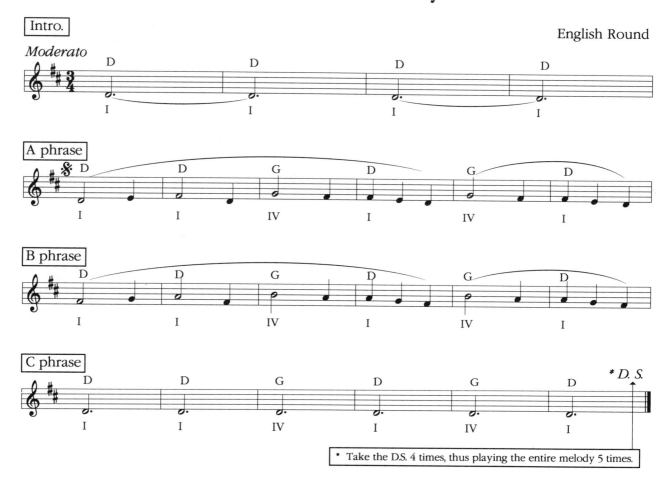

GAELIC WALTZ

Band: 6

Origin: Scotland

Melodic form: abcd (phrases)

Type of selection: Instrumental

Introduction: 4 macrobeats

Length: 2:06

Meter: Triple

Key or mode: G major

Major instrument(s): Violin, guitar

Tempo: 50 macrobeats per minute, 150 microbeats per minute

Repetitions of selection: 3

Music concepts

Steady beat, same/different phrases, macrobeat, identification of ♩. ♪ ♩ rhythm pattern, identification of waltz bass and arpeggiated accompaniment pattern

Movement concepts for dance

Macrobeat, pathways, directionality

Suggestions for use

With related books

Movement Plus Music, pp. 28, 31, 36

Foundations in Elementary Education: Music, pp. 90, 194, 195; also work with these key experiences in music:

- Moving to music
- Listening to and describing music
- Feeling and expressing steady beat
- Feeling and identifying meter

Foundations in Elementary Education: Movement, pp. 175, 211; also work with these key experiences in movement:

- Acting upon movement directions
- Feeling and expressing steady beat (macrobeat)
- Moving in sequences to a common beat (Level IIIB)

In activities

Rock to the macrobeat either in pairs or as a group, with long poles.

Move creatively with scarves.

Walk or skate to the macrobeat.

Lead slow dynamic movements for mirroring or reversal.

Folk dance

Teaching Movement & Dance: A Sequential Approach, p. 167

Video

Beginning Folk Dances Illustrated 4

Additional information

This beautiful melody is a favorite rocking selection with young children.

The dance is choreographed by Phyllis S. Weikart.

Melodic notation with primary chords identified

(see next page)

Gaelic Waltz

Scottish Melody

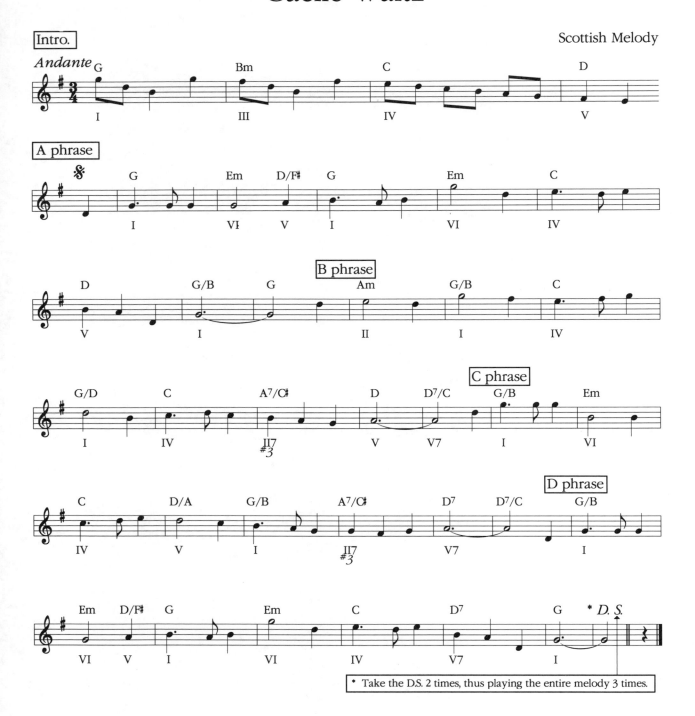

* Take the D.S. 2 times, thus playing the entire melody 3 times.

Band: 7

Origin: United States

Melodic form: AAABC

Type of selection: Instrumental

Introduction: 4 microbeats

Length: 2:33

Meter: Duple

Key or mode: G Mixolydian modality

Major instrument(s): Violin, guitar, pennywhistle, harmonica, bones, bongo drum

Tempo: 108 microbeats per minute

Repetitions of selection: 1

Music concepts

Steady beat; melodic echo; major/minor chord relationships of I to VI, IV to II, V$\sharp^3$ to VII chords; mode identification; melody fragment; melodic sequence; repeated rhythmic pattern

Suggestions for use

With related books

Movement Plus Music, p. 33

Foundations in Elementary Education: Music, work with these key experiences in music:

- Moving to music
- Listening to and describing music
- Feeling and expressing steady beat
- Developing melody
- Adding harmony

Foundations in Elementary Education: Movement, p. 262; also work with these key experiences in movement:

- Acting upon movement directions
- Moving in nonlocomotor ways
- Feeling and expressing steady beat
- Moving in sequences to a common beat

In activities

Create movement echo sequences.

Rock to the macrobeat.

Pass beanbags to the macrobeat.

Devise ball routines: alone, with a partner, or in small groups.

Jump rope.

Develop stick routines.

Prepare for mallet patterns on tonebar instruments.

Folk dance

None

Additional information

Echo is composed by Sandor Slomovits and performed by Gemini.

The echo is performed one octave higher than notated.

This is an interesting use of a melody fragment and sequence, as well as of a repeated rhythm pattern.

This is an interesting use of the G Mixolydian mode, which includes F natural with a consistent major dominant chord (D, F#, A).

Melodic notation with primary chords identified

(see next page)

Echo

American Melody
Composed by Sandor Slomovits

G Mixolydian mode

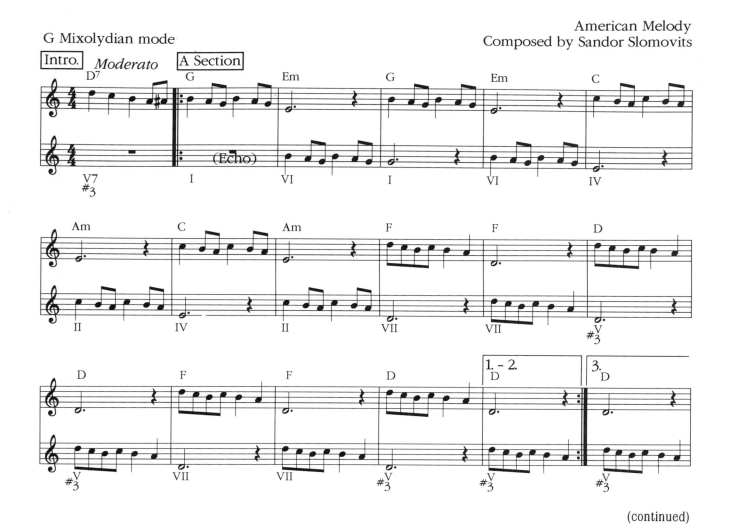

(continued)

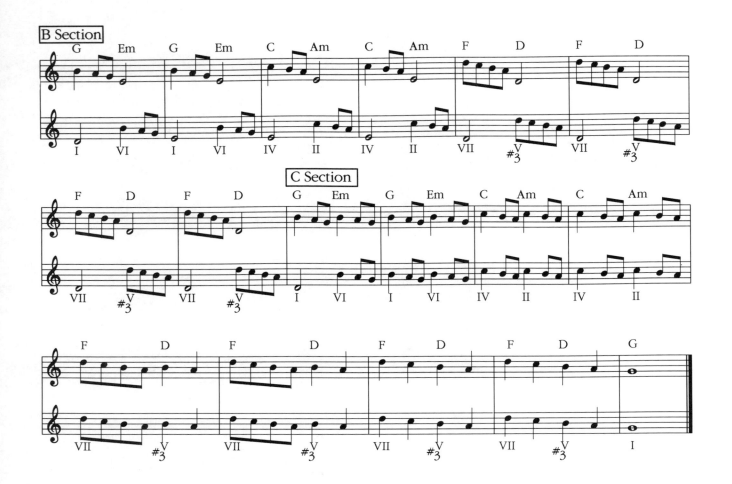

Band: 8	
Origin: Ireland	**Meter:** Duple
Melodic form: AB	**Key or mode:** C major
Type of selection: Instrumental	**Major instrument(s):** Pennywhistle, guitar
Introduction: None	**Tempo:** 102 microbeats per minute
Length: 2:32	**Repetitions of selection:** 2

Music concepts

Phrase; form; major/minor relationships; *rubato* tempo; arpeggiated bass accompaniment; chord pattern: I, V, IV, I; ornamentation: grace note, trill

Suggestions for use

With related books

Movement Plus Music, pp. 27, 31, 36

Foundations in Elementary Education: Music, work with these key experiences in music:

- Moving to music
- Labeling form
- Recognizing the expressive qualities of tempo
- Adding harmony

Foundations in Elementary Education: Movement, p. 312; also work with these key experiences in movement:

- Acting upon movement directions
- Moving in nonlocomotor ways
- Expressing creativity

In activities

Lead movements for mirroring.

Draw to music.

Move creatively with scarves, paper plates, or ribbon wands.

Folk dance

None

Additional information

Phrases 1, 2, and 4 are the same, therefore the chord pattern is also repeated.

Phrase 3 ends on an A minor chord, making the C major/A minor shared key signature relationship obvious.

During the second repetition, the guitar adds an arpeggiated bass accompaniment.

Melodic notation with primary chords identified

(see next page)

The Sally Gardens

A Section

Irish Melody

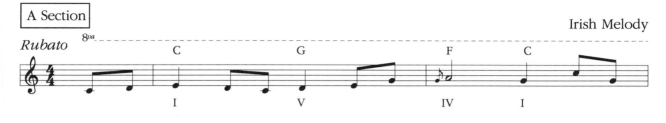

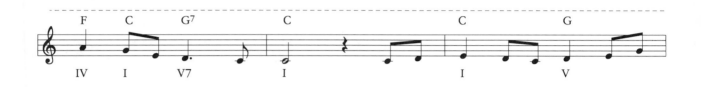

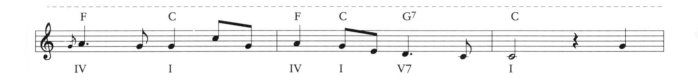

B Section

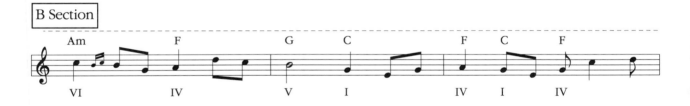

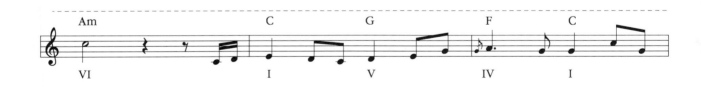

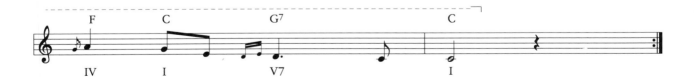

SOUTHWIND

Band: 9

Origin: Ireland

Melodic form: AB

Type of selection: Instrumental

Introduction: None

Length: 2:49

Meter: Triple

Key or mode: G major

Major instrument(s): Violin, guitar

Tempo: 36 macrobeats per minute

Repetitions of selection: 3

Music concepts

Steady macrobeat, phrase, arpeggiated accompaniment, primary chords used to complement the melody, AB form, rhythm pattern of ♩. ♪ ♩ , *ritardando* (end of last repetition)

Suggestions for use

With related books

Movement Plus Music, pp. 27, 31, 36, 38

Foundations in Elementary Education: Music, pp. 106, 134, 189; also work with these key experiences in music:

- Moving to music
- Feeling and expressing steady beat
- Labeling form
- Adding harmony

Foundations in Elementary Education: Movement, p. 197; also work with these key experiences in movement:

- Acting upon movement directions
- Moving in nonlocomotor ways
- Moving with objects
- Feeling and expressing steady beat

In activities

Rock, swing to the macrobeat.

Move creatively with scarves, ribbon wands, etc.

Lead the Stages of Movement for Responding, changing at the beginning of each phrase.

Lead movements for mirroring or visual copycat.

Pass beanbags or develop lumee stick routines.

Devise ball routines: pass/catch or bounce/catch with the macrobeat, bounce/catch with a partner (one partner throws on first beat, other partner catches on third beat).

Folk dance

None

Additional information

Sometimes a slight variation will be heard in further repetitions of the melody.

The guitar plays an arpeggiated accompaniment throughout.

During the third repetition, the guitarist adds a descending scale harmony.

Melodic notation with primary chords identified

(see next page)

Southwind

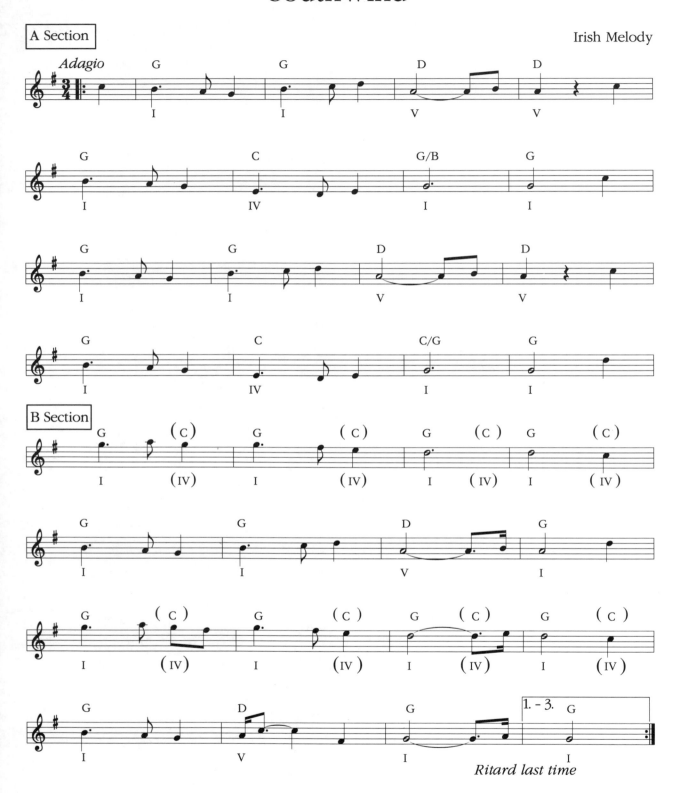

ARKANSAS TRAVELER/ SAILOR'S HORNPIPE/ TURKEY IN THE STRAW

Band: 10

Origin: British Isles

Melodic form:
Arkansas Traveler: AABB
Sailor's Hornpipe: AABB
Turkey in the Straw: AABB
Coda

Type of selection: Instrumental

Introduction: 4 microbeats

Length: 3:06

Meter: Duple

Key or mode:
Arkansas Traveler: D major
Sailor's Hornpipe: G major
Turkey in the Straw: C major

Major instrument(s): Banjo, violin, guitar

Tempo: 150 microbeats per minute

Repetitions of selection:
Arkansas Traveler: 3
Sailor's Hornpipe: 2
Turkey in the Straw: 2

Music concepts

Steady beat, *presto* tempo, form, phrase, melodic sections, medley, variation, rhythm patterns using sixteenth notes, *coda*

Movement concepts for dance

Directionality of forward, backward, in, out; personal/general space; moving in a circle

Suggestions for use

With related books

Foundations in Elementary Education: Music, work with these key experiences in music:

- ⚷ Moving to music
- ⚷ Listening to and describing movement
- ⚷ Feeling and expressing steady beat
- ⚷ Recognizing expressive qualities of tempo

- Labeling form
- Expressing rhythm

Foundations in Elementary Education: Movement, work with these key experiences in movement:

- Moving in nonlocomotor ways
- Moving in locomotor ways
- Feeling and expressing steady beat
- Moving in sequences to a common beat

In activities

Choose nonlocomotor ways to keep or lead steady beat (macrobeat).

Choose movement extensions using fast tempo.

Choreograph a square dance or longways set.

Choreograph a movement sequence for each selection in the medley.

Plan aerobic fitness routines.

Bounce and catch balls with the macrobeat.

Lead jogging parades.

Folk dance

Teaching Movement & Dance: A Sequential Approach (Big Circle Dance), p. 137

Additional information

The guitar plays a march bass accompaniment pattern throughout (for example, C, lower G, C, lower G).

During the second repetition of *Arkansas Traveler*, the violin plays the melody one octave higher and plays a melodic variation during the B section.

Melodic notation with primary chords identified

(see next page)

Arkansas Traveler

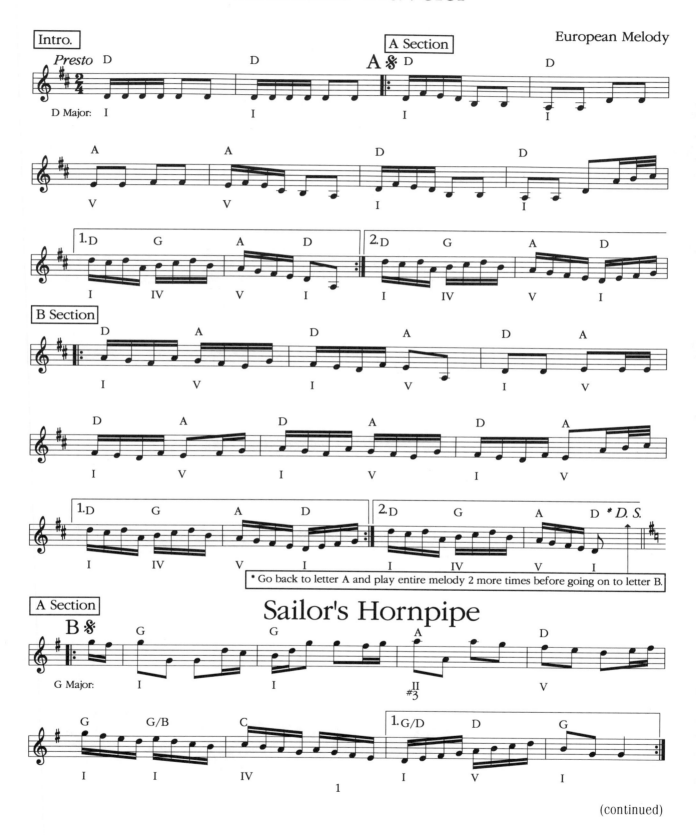

European Melody

* Go back to letter A and play entire melody 2 more times before going on to letter B.

Sailor's Hornpipe

(continued)

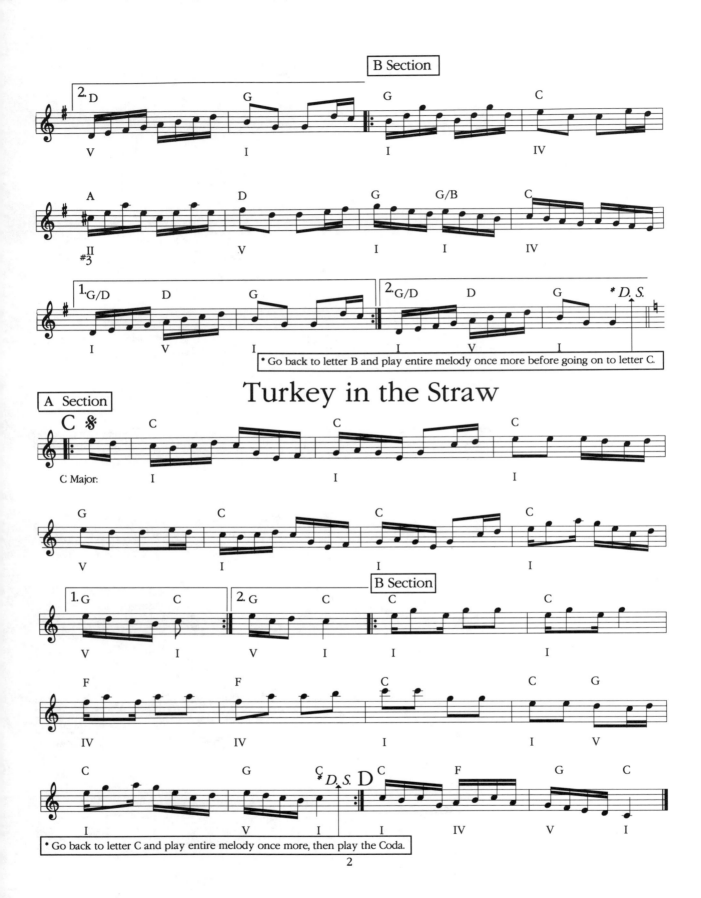

Turkey in the Straw

* Go back to letter B and play entire melody once more before going on to letter C.

* Go back to letter C and play entire melody once more, then play the Coda.

2

Band: 11

Origin: Ireland

Melodic form: AABB

Meter: Duple

Key or mode:
O'Keefe Slide: E Aeolian modality (natural minor)
Kerry Slide: D major

Type of selection: Instrumental

Major instrument(s): Pennywhistle, bones, violin, guitar, Irish drum

Introduction: 8 microbeats

Tempo: 128 microbeats per minute

Length: 3:09

Repetitions of selection:
O'Keefe Slide: 3
Kerry Slide: 3

Music concepts

Steady beat, microbeat divided into three, phrase, AABB form, major/minor relationships, repeated rhythm patterns, Aeolian mode identification, medley, *fermata,* D.S. (return to the sign, 𝄋)

Movement concepts for dance

Steady beat, clockwise/counterclockwise, alternating 4-beat pattern, do-si-do

Suggestions for use

With related books

Foundations in Elementary Education: Music, p. 234; also work with these key experiences in music:

- ⚷ Moving to music
- ⚷ Feeling and expressing steady beat
- ⚷ Labeling form
- ⚷ Feeling and identifying meter
- ⚷ Expressing rhythm

Foundations in Elementary Education: Movement, work with these key experiences in movement:

- Moving in nonlocomotor ways
- Moving in locomotor ways
- Feeling and expressing steady beat
- Moving in sequences to a common beat

In activities

Lead basic nonlocomotor movements to the music.

Gallop, slide, and skip to the music.

Rock to the macrobeat or walk to the microbeat.

Practice ball skills to music (toss/catch, bounce/catch, partner passing).

Create and perform nonlocomotor or locomotor movement maps to the music.

Lead parades.

Folk dance

Teaching Movement & Dance: A Sequential Approach (Big Circle Dance, Two-Part Dance, Irish Mixer), pp. 137, 142, 221

Additional information

In *O'Keefe Slide,* the pennywhistle is added on the second repetition; the violin and bones are used on the third repetition.

In *Kerry Slide,* the violin and bones are heard throughout.

The dance is choreographed by Phyllis S. Weikart.

Melodic notation with primary chords identified

(see next page)

O'Keefe Slide

E-Aeolian Mode

Irish Melody

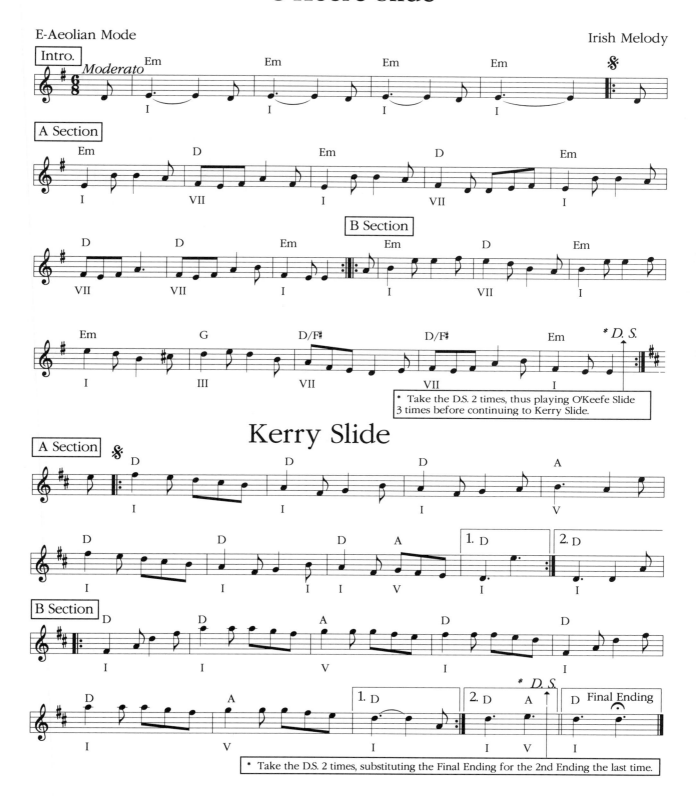

* Take the D.S. 2 times, thus playing O'Keefe Slide 3 times before continuing to Kerry Slide.

Kerry Slide

* Take the D.S. 2 times, substituting the Final Ending for the 2nd Ending the last time.

JOE CLARK MIXER (OLD JOE CLARK)

Band: 12

Origin: United States

Melodic form: AABB

Type of selection: Instrumental

Introduction: 8 microbeats

Length: 3:02

Meter: Duple

Key or mode: G Mixolydian modality

Major instrument(s): Harmonica, jaw harp, banjo, guitar

Tempo: 134 microbeats per minute

Repetitions of selection: 6

Music concepts

Steady beat; theme and variations; phrase; AABB form; repeated rhythm patterns of ♩♫ ♫♫ and ♩.♪ ♫♩ ; chord progression: I, VII, I (Mixolydian); identification of Mixolydian modality

Movement concepts for dance

Steady beat, clockwise/counterclockwise, alternating 4-beat pattern, do-si-do, directionality, partner mixer, hand-jive

Suggestions for use

With related books

Movement Plus Music, p. 25

Foundations in Elementary Education: Music, work with these key experiences in music:

- Moving to music
- Feeling and expressing steady beat
- Listening to and describing music
- Labeling form
- Expressing rhythm
- Adding harmony
- Responding to various types of music

Foundations in Elementary Education: Movement, p. 223; also work with these key experiences in movement:

- Moving in nonlocomotor ways

- Moving in locomotor ways
- Moving in integrated ways
- Feeling and expressing steady beat
- Moving in sequences to a common beat

In activities

Perform aerobic routines.

Develop marching routines.

Rock to the macrobeat with poles.

Choreograph progressive circle and square dances.

Play rhythm instruments to the steady beat.

Folk dance

Teaching Movement & Dance: A Sequential Approach, p. 250

Video

Beginning Folk Dances Illustrated 3

Additional information

1st repetition: The harmonica is predominant.

2nd repetition: At times the violin plays a melodic variation.

3rd repetition: The violin and harmonica play the variation.

4th repetition: The banjo is predominant for melody.

5th repetition: This is a slightly different variation; the jaw harp is added on the B section.

6th repetition: All instruments are used for richer sound.

The dance is choreographed by Phyllis S. Weikart.

Melodic notation with primary chords identified

(see next page)

Joe Clark Mixer

G Mixolydian Mode

American Melody

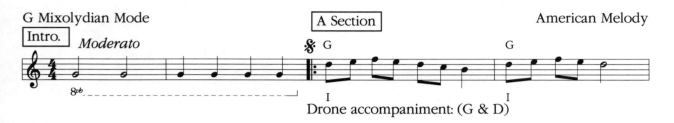

A Section

Drone accompaniment: (G & D)

B Section

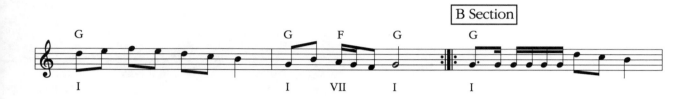

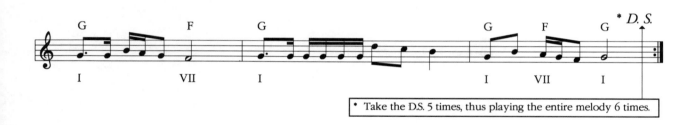

* D. S.

> * Take the D.S. 5 times, thus playing the entire melody 6 times.

NIGUN

Band: 13

Origin: United States

Melodic form: AABBCC

Meter: Duple

Key or mode:
Section A: E minor
Section B: C major
Section C: E minor

Type of selection: Instrumental

Introduction: 4 microbeats

Length: 2:09

Major instrument(s): Violin, guitar

Tempo: 118 microbeats per minute

Repetitions of selection: 5

Music concepts

Steady beat, repeated phrases, minor/major relationships, repeated rhythmic patterns, *moderato* tempo

Movement concepts for dance

Steady microbeat, pathways, directionality, recurring 2-beat locomotor sequences moving sideward, personal/general space

Suggestions for use

With related books

Movement Plus Music, p. 14

Foundations in Elementary Education: Music, p. 258; also work with these key experiences in music:

- Moving to music
- Feeling and expressing steady beat
- Feeling and identifying meter
- Expressing rhythm
- Responding to various types of music

Foundations in Elementary Education: Movement, work with these key experiences in movement:

- Acting upon movement directions

- Feeling and expressing steady beat
- Moving in sequences to a common beat

In activities

Using nonlocomotor action words, develop routines performed to the macrobeat.

March, jump, hop to the microbeat.

Use movement to show length of phrases.

Choreograph dances using the 3-part musical form.

Folk dance

Teaching Movement & Dance: A Sequential Approach, p. 162

Video

Beginning Folk Dances Illustrated 4

Additional information

Nigun (with its title meaning "wordless melody") is composed by Laszlo Slomovits and performed by Gemini in the style of the Eastern European Chassidic Jewish tradition.

The dance is choreographed by Phyllis S. Weikart.

Melodic notation with primary chords identified

(see next page)

Nigun

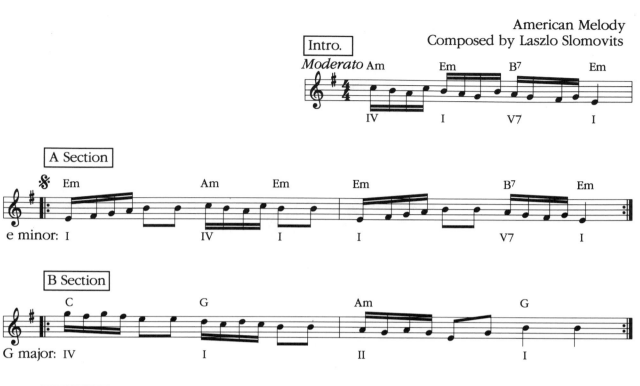

TE VE OREZ

Band: 14

Origin: Israel

Melodic form: ab (phrases)

Type of selection: Instrumental

Introduction: 8 microbeats

Length: 2:20

Meter: Duple

Key or mode:
C major 6 times
G major 6 times
D major 6 times

Major instrument(s): Piano, violin

Tempo: 132 microbeats per minute

Repetitions of selection: 18

Music concepts

Steady beat, repeated phrases, melodic sequence, major/minor relationship, *allegro* tempo, key changes to G major and D major

Movement concepts for dance

Steady microbeat; jog, slide, walk; directionality

Suggestions for use

With related books

Foundations in Elementary Education: Music, work with these key experiences in music:

- Moving to music
- Feeling and expressing steady beat
- Identifying tone color
- Developing melody
- Labeling form
- Feeling and identifying meter

Foundations in Elementary Education: Movement, pp. 192, 379; also work with these key experiences in movement:

- Acting upon movement directions
- Moving in nonlocomotor ways
- Moving in locomotor ways

- Feeling and expressing steady beat
- Moving in sequences to a common beat

In activities

Lead static Stages of Movement for Responding, changing every 8 microbeats.

Perform nonlocomotor movements to identify phrases.

Lead parades; pause to change leader every 32 microbeats.

Lead Levels I–IV of Beat Coordination.

Perform locomotor movements, changing the movement every 8 macrobeats.

Perform aerobic routines.

Folk dance

Teaching Movement & Dance: A Sequential Approach, p. 131

Additional information

Te Ve Orez is a mixer danced in trios. The center person of each trio moves to the new group.

The translation of *Te Ve Orez* is "tea and rice."

The first note of the melody in the new key is exactly one octave higher than the last note of the previous key.

Melodic notation with primary chords identified

(see next page)

Te Ve Orez

Israeli Melody

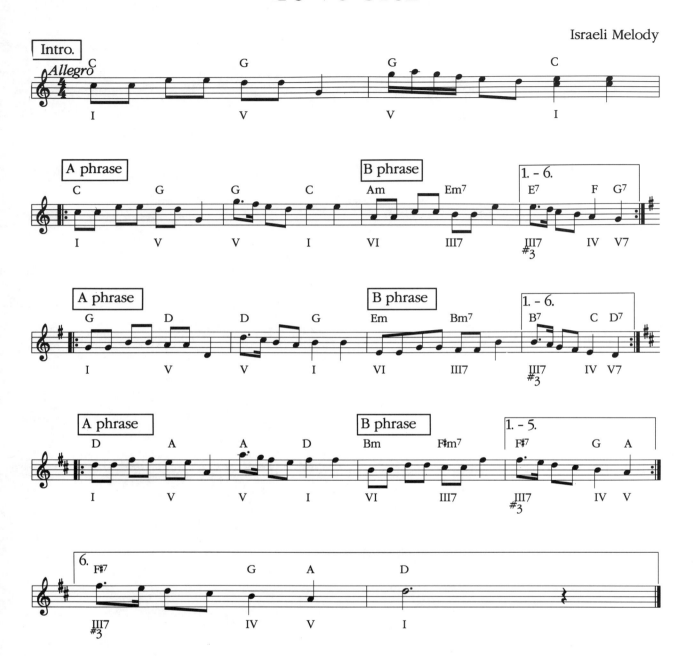

LES SALUTS

Band: 15

Origin: Quebec

Melodic form: AAB

Meter: Duple

Key or mode:
D major 2 times
G major 2 times
D major 3 times

Type of selection: Instrumental

Major instrument(s): Violin, guitar, pennywhistle

Introduction: 4 microbeats

Length: 2:28

Tempo: 132 microbeats per minute

Repetitions of selection: 7

Music concepts

Steady beat; *fermatas* of varying length; phrase; AAB form; chord identification: I, V, V⁷; key changes; microbeat divided into three

Movement concepts for dance

Steady microbeat walking, clockwise/counterclockwise directionality, balance on pauses

Suggestions for use

With related books

Foundations in Elementary Education: Music, work with these key experiences in music:

- ⊶ Moving to music
- ⊶ Feeling and expressing steady beat
- ⊶ Labeling form
- ⊶ Feeling and identifying meter

Foundations in Elementary Education: Movement, work with these key experiences in movement:

- ⊶ Moving in nonlocomotor ways
- ⊶ Moving in locomotor ways
- ⊶ Feeling and expressing steady beat (A sections of the music)

In activities

Lead locomotor movements on the A sections and nonlocomotor movements on the B sections of the music, with a pause on each *fermata.*

Lead parades, changing leader on the *fermata.*

Play rhythm instruments to the steady beat.

Perform two different nonlocomotor movements during the A sections, one locomotor movement during the B sections, and stop in a balanced position on the *fermata.*

Folk dance

Teaching Movement & Dance: A Sequential Approach, p. 126

Additional information

Les Saluts is a French-Canadian children's dance.

Repetitions 3 and 4 are played in the key of G major.

There is no *fermata* on the seventh (last) repetition.

Melodic notation with primary chords identified

(see next page)

Les Saluts

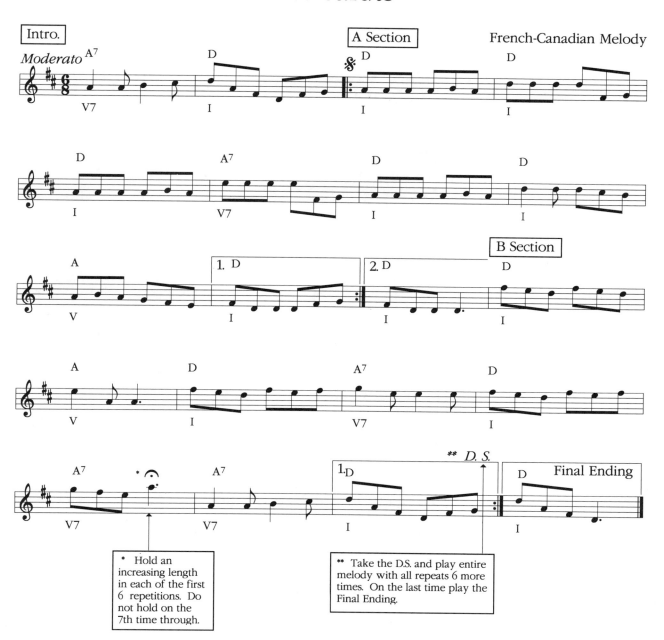

* Hold an increasing length in each of the first 6 repetitions. Do not hold on the 7th time through.

** Take the D.S. and play entire melody with all repeats 6 more times. On the last time play the Final Ending.

COBBLER'S REEL/ GASPÉ REEL

Band: 16

Origin: Quebec

Meter: Duple

Melodic form:
Cobbler's Reel: ABABA
Gaspé Reel: ABABAB

Key or mode:
Cobbler's Reel: G major
Gaspé Reel: D major

Type of selection: Instrumental

Major instrument(s): Violin, guitar, bones

Introduction: 3 microbeats plus pickup

Tempo: 128 microbeats per minute

Length: 2:55

Repetitions of selection:
Cobbler's Reel: 2½
Gaspé Reel: 3

Music concepts

Steady beat; phrase; AB form; medley; key change; repeated chord progression: I, V, I, V *(Cobbler's)*; I, V⁷, I, V⁷ *(Gaspé)*; repeated rhythmic patterns using ♪♫ ♫♫ .

Movement concepts for dance

Steady microbeat walking, directionality, single circle, personal and general space, recurring 2-beat nonlocomotor movement sequences

Suggestions for use

With related books

Movement Plus Music, p. 25

Foundations in Elementary Education: Music, work with these key experiences in music:

- ⟳ Moving to music
- ⟳ Feeling and expressing steady beat
- ⟳ Developing melody
- ⟳ Labeling form
- ⟳ Feeling and identifying meter

- Adding harmony
- Choreographing movement sequences

Foundations in Elementary Education: Movement, p. 193; also work with these key experiences in movement:

- Acting upon movement directions
- Moving in nonlocomotor ways
- Moving in locomotor ways
- Moving with objects
- Moving in sequences to a common beat

In activities

Form parades in which students walk the microbeat.

Lead Stages of Movement for Responding.

Move in pathways (straight, curved, zigzag) for each section of the music.

Show spatial relationships and extensions of locomotor movement.

Develop aerobic routines.

Pass beanbags and perform lumee stick routines.

Lead Levels I–VI of Beat Coordination.

Folk dance

Teaching Movement & Dance: A Sequential Approach (Big Circle Dance), p. 137

Additional information

Recurring and alternating 2- and 4-beat sequences and dance steps can make the *Big Circle Dance* useful as a warm-up for more experienced dancers.

Melodic notation with primary chords identified

(see next page)

Cobbler's Reel

French-Canadian Melody

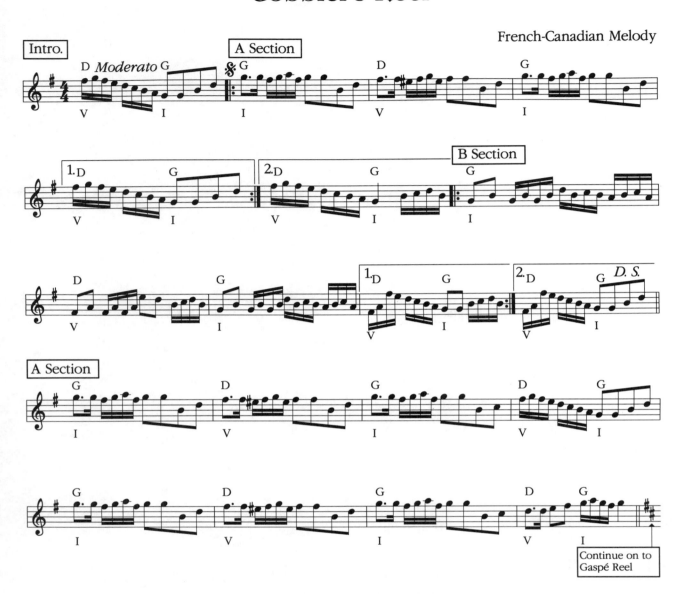

Continue on to
Gaspé Reel

Gaspé Reel

French-Canadian Melody

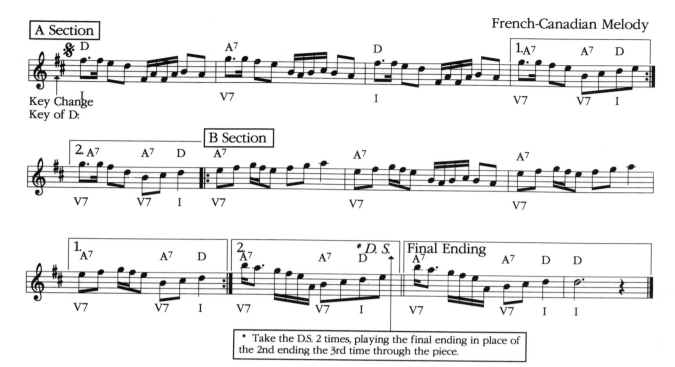

* Take the D.S. 2 times, playing the final ending in place of the 2nd ending the 3rd time through the piece.